My pregnancy Guide

What should I expect during your pregnancy?

Dr Miller. S.Wick

Disclaimer

Table of Contents

Title

Disclaimer

Table of Contents

Introduction

Chapter One

What exactly is pregnancy?

Early warning signs

Chapter Two

Stages in Pregnancy

Early development

Expected Symptoms

Chapter Three

Precautions and Tips

Precautions

Complications

Suggestions for reducing discomfort

What will I do if I go into labor?

Conclusion

Introduction

One of tge most exciting things that can occur to you is having a baby. But maybe you're nervous too. When it's your first baby, it's hard to know what to expect. Your mother, co-workers, friends, and loved ones could all give you advice. And then information on the internet is available, likewise in magazines and books. Sometimes it can feel overwhelming, and it's hard to know who's right when people say different things.

The best way to prepare for both motherhood and pregnancy is to educate yourself. In this guide to what to expect during pregnancy, we will review and understand the trimesters and the changes you can expect as your pregnancy progresses. You will also learn how to take care of your health and that of your baby and how to prepare for labor and delivery. You can never be 100% sure you're pregnant until you take a home pregnancy test or blood test at your obstetrician's office. To get the best results, take the test after you miss your period. Missing your period doesn't necessarily mean you're pregnant, but it's one of the main signs that you might be pregnant.

To count the duration of a pregnancy, we start from the first day of your last period until the 37th–40th day of the month. the week. These 37 to 40 weeks are then divided into three trimesters, each lasting 13 weeks.

The first trimester starts with the first week from the first day of your last period until the 13th week. During the first trimester, although your pregnancy may not manifest, your body goes through many internal changes as it tries to adjust to the growing fetus.

To make this guide easier to read and complete, we have divided each quarter into different forms for better understanding.

Chapter One

What exactly is pregnancy?

Pregnancy is the period during which one or more offspring (gestates) develop inside a woman's womb.

Twins are one example of multiple pregnancies that result in multiple children.

In most cases, sexual activity results in pregnancy, however assisted reproductive technology procedures can also result in pregnancy. Live birth, spontaneous miscarriage, induced miscarriage, or stillbirth are the possible outcomes of pregnancy.

Pregnancy is a 9-month period during which an unborn baby develops in the uterus. Missed menstruation is usually the first sign of pregnancy, but there are others.

Most pregnancies last about 280 days or approximately 40 weeks. A pregnancy calculator can assist in predicting when a baby will be born.

Early warning signs

Recognizing Early Warning Signs

A missed menstrual cycle is one of the most common early signs of pregnancy. The American Pregnancy Association reports that 29% of pregnant women reported this as their first sign of pregnancy. Other than a missed period, signs of pregnancy may appear as early as the first few weeks of conception.

With or without vomiting, nausea
Tiredness Dizziness
Tenderness in the breasts, frequent urination as a result of hormonal changes, increased blood flow through the kidneys with light implantation spotting or bleeding, fatigue

Not all pregnant women have the same symptoms, and some have no symptoms at all.

A pregnancy test looks for the hormone human chorionic gonadotropin (HCG) in the blood or urine. HCG is present only a few days after conception.

The hormone levels are low at the start of pregnancy and gradually rise. A high level of HCG can indicate multiple pregnancies, such as when a woman is expecting twins or triplets.

If a pregnancy test results in a positive result, a person can undergo an abdominal or transvaginal ultrasound scan.

Chapter Two

Stages in Pregnancy

What Is the First Trimester of Pregnancy? (Week 1–13)

The first trimester is the most advanced stage of pregnancy. It begins on the first day of your last period, even before you're pregnant, and lasts until the end of the 13th week. It's an amazing time with more changes for you and your baby. Knowing what to expect will assist you in preparing for the months ahead. During the first three months, some women glow with good health, while others are miserable.

The first trimester lasts 13 weeks and includes periods of ovulation and conception.

Conception occurs when male sperm penetrates and fertilizes a female egg. After ovulation, this usually occurs in the female's fallopian tube. The result is a zygote (a sperm-egg cell hybrid).

Following that, the zygote immediately begins to divide, forming a cluster of cells known as an embryo.

After dividing and growing, the embryo attaches to the uterine wall and produces root-like veins known as villi. This is known as implantation.
Occasionally, the embryo implants somewhere other than the uterine lining, most commonly in the fallopian tube. This causes an ectopic pregnancy.

The villi ensure that the embryo is anchored to the uterine lining when it implants normally. They will eventually develop into the placenta, which feeds and protects the embryo as it develops, providing oxygen and nutrition while excreting waste.

Early development

The embryo then begins to grow rapidly. The heart, spinal cord, brain, and gastrointestinal tract are the first to develop. The placenta begins to develop. More structures and organs develop over time. A doctor may be able to detect a heartbeat by week 6.

By week 7, the majority of vital organs have formed. By week 8, the embryo contains everything that adult humans have both inside and outside, but in a much smaller form.

By week 9, the embryo has developed into a fetus and is growing inside the uterus, surrounded by amniotic fluid. This is the "water" that "breaks" just before the baby is born. The fetus will be about 3 inches long and weigh about 1 ounce (oz) by the end of this stage.

Expected Symptoms

The symptoms of pregnancy will most likely be similar to those seen in the early stages of the first 13 weeks, but they may worsen as time goes on.

Here are some of the changes that you may notice, what they actually mean, and which of these signs should warrant you to contact your doctor. signs should prompt you to contact your doctor.

Bleeding. Approximately 25% of pregnant women experience minor bleeding during the first trimester. Light spotting early in pregnancy may indicate that the fertilized embryo has been implanted in your uterus. If you experience severe bleeding, cramping, or sharp pain in your abdomen, contact a doctor, or sharp pain in your stomach. These could be symptoms of a miscarriage or an ectopic pregnancy (a pregnancy in which the uterus does not develop normally where the embryo implants outside the uterus).

Tenderness in the breasts

One of the first signs of pregnancy is sore breasts. These are caused by changes in the hormone which prepare your milk ducts to feed your baby. Your breast will most likely to be sore throughout the first trimester. Wearing a support bra and going up a bra size (or more) can make you feel more comfortable. It won't be possible for you to return to your normal bra size until your baby has finished nursing.

Constipation High levels of the hormone progesterone slow down the muscle contractions that normally move food through your system during pregnancy. Add in the extra iron from your prenatal vitamin, and the result is uncomfortable constipation and gas that can last for days. Consume more fiber and drink more fluids to keep things moving smoothly. Physical activity can also be beneficial.

If constipation is causing you problems, consult your doctor about which mild laxatives or stool softeners are safe to use during pregnancy.

Discharge

Early in your pregnancy, you may notice a thin, milky white discharge (called leukorrhea). Wear a panty liner if it makes you feel more comfortable, but don't use a tampon because it may introduce gems into your vagina. Contact a doctor if you notice that the discharge smells strong, or is green or yellow, or has a large amount of clear discharge.

Fatigue

Your body is putting more efforts to aid a growing baby. This means you'll tire more quickly than usual. Take a rest as needed during the day Check to see if you're getting enough iron. Too little can cause anemia, which can make you tired even more.

Food preferences and dislikes

Although you might not want a bowl of mint chip ice cream with dill pickles, as the adage goes, your tastes can change while pregnant. Food cravings affect more than 60% of pregnant women. More than 50% of the population dislikes certain foods. Cravings are acceptable as long as you eat healthy, low-calorie foods the majority of the time. The only exception is Pica, a craving for nonfoods such as clay, dirt, and laundry starch that can be harmful to you and your baby. Contact your doctor if you have cravings of this type.

I pee a lot.

Although your baby is still small, your uterus is expanding and putting pressure on your bladder. As a result, you may feel compelled to use the restroom regularly. Never stop drinking fluids; your body needs them. However, limit caffeine (which stimulates your bladder), especially before bedtime. Respond when nature calls as soon as possibleDon't keep it bottled up.

Gastric acid

During pregnancy, your body produces more progesterone hormone. Relax smooth muscles, such as the muscle ring in the lower esophagus, the tube that connects the mouth and stomach. These muscles normally hold food and acids in the stomach. When they become loose, you can have acid reflux, also known as heartburn. To avoid the burn, eat a few small meals throughout the day. Do not lie immediately after eating. Avoid fatty, spicy, and acidic foods (such as citrus fruits). Try to raise the pillows a bit when you sleep.

My mood swings. Increased fatigue and shifting hormones can send you on an emotional roller coaster, taking you from happy to unhappy or hopeful to scared in seconds. It's okay to cry, but if you're feeling overwhelmed, try to find an understanding ear. You can talk to your partner, a friend, a family member, or even a professional.

Morning sickness Nausea is one of the most common pregnancy complaints. Up to 85% of pregnant women are affected. It is the result of hormonal changes in your body and can last throughout the first trimester. For some pregnant women, the nausea is mild. Others can't start the day without throwing up.

Nausea usually gets worse in the morning (hence the name "morning sickness"). To calm nausea, try eating small, bland, or protein-rich snacks (crackers, meat, or cheese) and drinking water, clear fruit juice (apple juice), or ginger ale. You may also want to do this before you get out of bed. Avoid all foods that make your stomach feel nauseous. Nausea alone isn't something to worry about, but if it's severe or just doesn't go away, it can affect the amount of nourishment your baby gets. Call your doctor if you can't stop vomiting or withhold food.

gaining weight. Pregnancy is one of the few times in a woman's life when gaining weight is considered healthy, but don't go overboard. You should gain 3-6 pounds during the first trimester (your doctor may advise you to increase or decrease weight gain if you started your pregnancy underweight or overweight). Even if you have a companion, you don't eat for two. You only need about 150 extra calories per day during the first trimester. Get those calories the healthy way by increasing your intake of fruits and vegetables, milk, whole grain bread, and lean meats.

Weeks 13-28

During the second trimester, the fetus develops fluff, a type of fine hair on the head. It also begins sucking and creating fingerprints.

Sweat glands, brows, eyelashes, and eyes form. The brain, nervous system, and other vital organs are still growing. A fetus born at week 22 may be able to survive with medical assistance. By week 28, the fetus will weigh approximately 214 pounds and be 14 inches long.

The second trimester is when most women report feeling better. Often, nausea and fatigue end or are less severe during the first trimester. The second quarter, on the other hand, brings many other physical changes, such as:
Sensitive breasts should decrease at this point, but will likely grow as a result of milk production preparation. You might require a support bra.

Weight gain and an expanding stomach: When the belly begins to expand during the second trimester, a normal weight gain is 3-4 pounds per month. If you were previously overweight, your doctor or midwife can warn you about the weight gain.

Discharge from the cervix.

Braxton Hicks contractions occur when your uterus begins to contract in preparation for the baby and can begin as early as the second trimester. They are typically weak and painless. Consult your doctor if the pain worsens to ensure that you are not having a premature birth.

Leg cramps—These typically occur at night and can worsen as your pregnancy progresses.

Kidney and Bladder Infections: Contact a doctor if the swelling is sudden or severe, or if the itching is accompanied by vomiting, nausea, jaundice, fatigue, or loss of appetite. These symptoms could indicate preeclampsia or a liver problem.

Nausea usually goes away, and energy levels rise. Some people may continue to feel uneasy. Back pain, carpal tunnel syndrome, itchy palms and feet, and swelling of the face, fingers, or ankles are examples.
Some people may also develop skin discoloration and stretch marks.

Weeks 29–40

The third trimester lasts from week 29 to week 40, when the baby is born. The fetus will grow significantly in size during the first few weeks of this period. Even if his lungs are still developing, he will begin to make rhythmic breathing movements with them.

The bones are fully developed but still soft at this point. The eyelids lift. After week 33, the fetus typically turns upside down in preparation for birth. She'll keep gaining weight and losing her fluffy hair. You've made it this far, and your baby's arrival is just a few weeks away! But first, here are some ideas:

Back Pain: You are carrying a lot more weight than your body is used to right now. Back pain can result from the extra weight putting pressure on your back.

Sleeping difficulties: It can be difficult to sleep comfortably during the final weeks of pregnancy. One suggestion is to sleep on your side with a pillow between your legs.

Frequent urination is caused by bladder pressure as the fetus pushes against the stomach.

Bleeding: Do not be alarmed if you notice bleeding. Call your doctor and have him examine you to ensure there is nothing seriously wrong. Constipation and heartburn

Hemorrhoids

Swelling of the feet

Shortness of breath when the baby presses on the diaphragm

Some people may notice that their breasts are losing colostrum, a substance produced by the body in preparation for milk production. Premature labor can also happen days or weeks before the due date. These contractions are known as Braxton Hicks. They are not indicative of labor.

Chapter 3:

Precautions and Tips

Prenatal visits and care

During pregnancy, a woman will be monitored and tested regularly to ensure that the baby develops normally.

The initial visit

The first appointment is usually scheduled around the eighth week of pregnancy. An ultrasound, a Pap smear, or cervical cultures can be used to confirm a person's pregnancy. If there are multiple pregnancies, the ultrasound will reveal them.

In addition, the doctor will take a detailed medical history and conduct a physical examination. These procedures include taking a person's blood pressure and performing a urine test to look for signs of infection and other abnormalities. Another aspect of the first visit is sending a pregnant woman for a blood test to determine her blood type and to screen for diseases such as HIV and Hepatitis. A doctor can also check for a variety of genetic disorders that can harm the developing embryo.

At this point, the doctor will answer any questions the patient has and make recommendations on safe foods to eat while pregnant, prenatal vitamins, exercise while pregnant, safe medications to take while pregnant, and other topics. Further visits

A pregnant woman can expect to see a doctor once a month for the first 28 weeks after her first visit. A person comes every two weeks between the 28th and the 36th week. Visits become weekly from week 36 until birth.

The doctor may do the following during subsequent visits:

- Taking a pregnant woman's blood pressure

Calculate a pregnant woman's weight gain.

- Measure the abdomen to see how the fetus is developing as the pregnancy progresses.
- Examine the baby's position in preparation for birth.
- Perform additional blood or urine tests.
- Perform additional ultrasounds.

Throughout their pregnancy, most pregnant women will require several checkups. Some people may require additional tests if they are pregnant at high risk or have other medical conditions.

The following are the most common tests:

Between the 11th and 14th weeks of pregnancy, women are screened for chromosomal disorders such as Down syndrome and trisomy 18, as well as heart defects.

20-week ultrasound: Around the 20th week of pregnancy, many pregnant women have an ultrasound to check fetal development. The doctor examines the fetus for abnormalities and can provide the fetus's gender upon request. During a pregnancy exam, a pregnant woman may be required to take a urine test to rule out conditions such as urinary tract infections, diabetes, or preeclampsia.

Blood sugar test: Between the 26th and 28th week, this test checks for gestational diabetes. To determine blood sugar, a person should drink a sugary drink and wait an hour.

Group B strep test: During weeks 36 and 37, this test looks for bacteria that can be passed to babies during birth and cause a serious infection.

Precautions

During pregnancy, doctors advise pregnant women to keep an eye out for or avoid a variety of things. Tobacco use raises the risk of premature labor and birth defects.

Alcohol: There is no such thing as a safe amount of alcohol to consume during pregnancy. Alcohol consumption puts the baby at risk for birth defects and fetal alcohol syndrome. Marijuana and other drugs increase the risk of complications during pregnancy and birth defects in the baby.

Overheating: Excessive heat raises the risk of neural tube defects. Pregnant women should exercise caution in hot weather and treat fevers as soon as possible.

Pregnant women should avoid eating high-mercury fish like bigeye tuna or king mackerel. Pregnant women should avoid eating raw vegetables and meat, unpasteurized soft cheeses, deli meats, cabbage, and prepared salads such as chicken salad, to reduce their risk of contracting bacterial infections that can harm the fetus, such as salmonella and listeriosis.

Certain medications: Not all medications, both over-the-counter and prescription, can be taken safely during pregnancy. Some medications may not be safe to take until week 13. Before taking any medication, a person should consult with their doctor.

Soil: Infection can be transmitted through the soil and some animal feces. Toxoplasmosis caused by cat feces, for example, can be fatal to a fetus. Wear gloves and wash your hands thoroughly before and after gardening or changing the kitty litter. Caffeine: According to the American College of Obstetricians and Gynecologists, pregnant women should consume no more than 200 mg of caffeine per day.

Complications

Pregnant women may experience additional symptoms that necessitate medical attention in addition to the usual pregnancy symptoms. This includes dental issues, urinary tract infections, and anemia. Basic medical treatments are available for these types of conditions.

However, complications can be serious in some cases. Here are some examples:

The medical word for high blood pressure is **hypertension**. High blood pressure puts a pregnant woman at risk of preeclampsia, so she will need to be monitored and may require medication to control it.

Preeclampsia occurs when a pregnant woman's high blood pressure reduces the blood supply to the fetus. If the condition is not treated promptly, the person may develop eclampsia, which can cause seizures and lead to death.

Gestational diabetes occurs when a person who did not previously have diabetes develops it during pregnancy. If it is not controlled by doctors, it can lead to high blood pressure, which can lead to preeclampsia.

If a pregnant woman contracts an infection, including some sexually transmitted infections (STIs), she may experience miscarriage, preterm labor, and stillbirth. The baby could be at risk for birth defects.

Placenta previa occurs when the placenta covers part or all of the cervix, the passage through which the baby exits the uterus. This problem may be resolved on its own. If not, a cesarean section will be required.

Suggestions for reducing discomfort

Although it is not always possible to avoid the unpleasant symptoms of pregnancy, the following strategies may be beneficial:

Maintain physical activity: exercise to keep your general health and weight in check, as well as to help with labor and delivery. Walking and swimming are frequently appropriate activities. Doctors advise against playing contact sports.

Keep a healthy weight: "Eating for two" does not imply that a pregnant woman should eat twice as much. Although weight gain during pregnancy is normal, doctors advise pregnant women to gain 2-4 pounds in the first trimester and another 3-4 pounds in the second and third trimesters. A person with a high body mass index (BMI) should see a doctor because they may be at risk of developing diabetes.

Eat a healthy and balanced diet, which includes plenty of fruits, vegetables, and whole grains in reasonable portions.

Take vitamins and supplements exactly as directed by your doctor. Doctors frequently recommend folic acid, calcium, vitamin D, and a variety of other supplements. Some vitamins, such as vitamin A, may be harmful to a baby if consumed in excessive amounts. Prenatal vitamins can be purchased at any pharmacy or online.

Drink plenty of fluids. Pregnant women should drink at least 2 liters of fluid per day, preferably water.

Your body will prepare for the birth of your baby (stage one), deliver the baby (stage two), and deliver the placenta during the three stages of labor. Your body will use contractions to dilate and efface your cervix throughout labor.

How does labor function?

Your body will begin to prepare for labor and delivery as your pregnancy comes to an end. This is the procedure by which your child will be born. Labor is frequently unique to each individual. Some have quick labor, while others have long, difficult labor. Others may have labor that stalls or stops, necessitating medical intervention.

Early work

Labor typically lasts 12 to 24 hours for a first birth and eight to ten hours for subsequent births.

You will go through three stages of labor during this time. The first stage of labor is usually the longest, lasting from the time you go into labor until your cervix opens. Early labor refers to the beginning of this stage. Early labor is defined as dilating between 0 and 6 centimeters.

Active work

As you progress and your contractions become stronger, you will enter the second stage of labor, known as active labor. Active labor is defined as dilation of 6 to 8 centimeters, followed by dilation of 8 to 10 centimeters. During active labor, your contractions will become stronger, and your cervix will quickly open. When you reach the second stage of labor, this is the stage of labor in which you will give birth to your baby.

Afterbirth

When the placenta is delivered is the third stage. This is also known as afterbirth.

Your body prepares for childbirth during these stages by going through dilation and effacement.

Dilation is the process by which your cervix stretches and opens to allow for the birth of your baby. Between 1 to 10 centimeters are used to measure dilation. Throughout your labor, your provider will perform a vaginal exam to determine how dilated you are. In the second stage of labor, you will be 10 centimeters dilated for the delivery of your baby.

Effacement: During labor, the cervix not only stretches but also thins. Cervical shortening and thinning are measured in percentages. During your labor, you will progress from 0% to 100% effacement.

Consider your cervix to be a round doorway that must stretch outward and become thinner before your baby can pass through. The contraction causes this stretching and thinning. Contractions can be described as anything from uncomfortable period cramps to a painful tightening of your abdomen. You may also experience a dull ache in your back and lower abdomen, as well as pelvic pressure.

When you have a contraction, your uterine muscles tighten at regular intervals to dilate and efface (open and thin) your cervix. Your abdomen hardens during contractions. Your uterus relaxes and your abdomen softens between contractions. Even though they can be uncomfortable, each contraction helps you progress through your labor.

What will I do if I go into labor?

When you're truly in labour, it can be difficult to tell sometimes. Other symptoms or irregular practice contractions (called Braxton Hicks contractions) may be misinterpreted as true labor by first-time parents in particular. True labor follows a pattern and advances steadily over time.

You'll notice a pattern in your contractions when you're in true labor. Instead of the irregular Braxton Hicks contractions that appeared and then disappeared at random during your pregnancy, these contractions will continue for an extended period. When you are in true labor, you should look for three things.

Frequency: How frequently do your contractions occur?

Keep track of them in a journal or on your phone with a labor app to ensure they arrive at regular intervals.

Duration (How long does each of your contractions last)?

Your contractions will last longer and longer as your labor progresses. Keep a stopwatch, a clock, or the timer on your phone handy to record the length of each contraction.

Intensity: (Are your contractions becoming more intense)?

Contractions can become stronger and more intense as you progress through the stages of labor. Observe how your contractions feel over time.

Is there anything indicating that I will go into labor soon?

Many women exhibit several pre-labor symptoms, which may indicate that labor will begin soon. These are some examples of labor signs:

- Backaches
- Diarrhea
- loss of weight.
- Nesting (cleaning and organizing your home).
- Nobody knows for certain what causes labor to begin, but several hormonal and physical changes may indicate the start of labor.

Braxton Hick's contractions are what they sound like. Braxton Hicks contractions, also known as practice contractions, are irregular contractions that do not cause cervical change. Consider them a practice run for the real thing. They can start at the end of your pregnancy and fool people into thinking you're in labor. This is known as "false labor."

Braxton Hicks contractions are characterized by a sudden, sharp tightening of your abdominal muscles. Even though this feels very similar to a contraction, Braxton Hick's contractions do not follow a pattern or progress over time.

They may also come to a halt if you lie down or relax. Keep a record of any practice contractions that you encounter. The best way to tell the difference between true and false labor is to write it down.

What exactly is lightning?

The method by which your child lowers or settles into your pelvis is known as "lighting. This can happen months or hours before labor. When this occurs, you may notice an increase in lower back pain. Because your uterus rests more heavily on your bladder after lightening, you may feel the need to urinate more frequently. You may notice that you aren't out of breath after your baby is born.

What exactly is the mucus plug, and what does it indicate when it falls out?

A plug is a thick piece of mucus that blocks the cervical opening during pregnancy. This plug seals off your uterus from the birth canal and the outside world, preventing bacteria from entering your uterus. The mucus is expelled into your vagina when your cervix softens, thins, and opens. Every mucus plug will be different. The mucus plug can be any of the following colors:

- Clear.
- Pink
- A little bloody.

Labor may begin soon after you lose your mucus plug, or it may begin several weeks later.

How should my contractions be timed?

It's critical to keep track of your contractions once you're in labor. Your doctor will want to know how long your contractions last (duration), how frequently they occur (frequency), and how intense they are. When timing your contractions, you'll need a way to record each one—pen and paper or an app on your phone—as well as a timer or clock. Keep track of each contraction from beginning to end, as well as the time between each contraction. This second measurement will provide your provider with information about the frequency of your contractions.

It can be difficult to keep track of the strength of your contractions. From person to person, this varies tremendously.

Recording when you can't walk, talk, or laugh during contractions is a simple way to keep track of the intensity of your contractions.

There are also methods for dealing with labor discomforts at home or without medication, such as:

- Take a walk, go shopping, or watch a movie to distract yourself.
- Take a hot shower or a soak at a spa. If your water bag has broken, consult your doctor about whether you should take a tub bath.
- Place your feet on a birth ball.
- Play some music.
- Turn off the lights.
- Make use of aromatherapy.
- Get yourself a massage.
- Maintain your upright posture. This can aid your baby's descent and rotation.
- If it's late at night, try to sleep. You'll want to conserve energy before going into active labor and delivery.

When my water breaks, how will I know?

You've probably heard the phrase "my water broke." This is the rupture of your amniotic membrane. Your baby is contained within a fluid-filled sac known as "your bag of water" during pregnancy. When this membrane ruptures, you may notice a sudden gush or trickle of fluid. This experience, like many aspects of labor and childbirth, can be unique to each individual. The fluid is usually odorless and clear, but it can also be straw-colored.

This, unlike the urine leakage that some pregnant women experience, will not stop. Amniotic fluid will frequently continue to leak.

If your water breaks, contact your doctor. Tell your provider when your water broke, how much water came out (trickle or gush), the color of the fluid, and the odor. Tampons should not be used if your water has broken. Your labor may begin immediately after your water breaks. Some women are already in labor when their water breaks, whereas others do not enter the first stage of labor for some time after their water breaks.

When should I contact my doctor or go to the hospital?
When you start having regular contractions, call your provider to discuss when you should go to the hospital. Some women can stay at home during the early stages of labor. Others may need to arrive sooner.

Your doctor should be contacted if you believe your water has broken. This could be a sudden gush of fluid or a steady trickle of fluid.
Are you bleeding? (more than spotting).
Very painful contractions have been coming every five minutes, lasting one minute, and have been going on for an hour.

What happens once I arrive at the hospital?

When you arrive at the hospital, check in at the labor and delivery desk. The majority of people will be seen in a triage room first. This is a requirement for admission. It is usually advised that you only bring one person to the triage room.

You will be taken from the triage room to the labor, delivery, and recovery (LDR) room. You will be required to dress in a hospital gown. Your heart rate, blood pressure, and temperature will be measured. For a short period, an external fetal monitor will be placed on your abdomen to check for uterine contractions and measure your baby's heart rate. Your doctor will also examine your cervix to see how far your labor has progressed. An intravenous (IV) line may be inserted into a vein in your arm to deliver fluids and medications.

What does it mean to have induced labor?
Labor does not always begin or progress as it should. In these cases, your provider may discuss

inducing labor with you. This is a medical procedure in which your healthcare provider initiates labor. This could occur if you:

- You've passed your deadline.
- Have health issues such as high blood pressure, preeclampsia, infection, or diabetes.
- Your water broke but labor did not begin.
- Amniotic fluid levels are low.

Your labor can be accelerated or induced in a variety of ways. Depending on your health, your provider will advise you on the best and safest option. To induce labor, use the following methods:

Medications (oxytocin) are administered via IV (directly into your veins). Rupturing your amniotic sac (water). Separating the amniotic membrane (the sac of fluid inside your uterus containing the baby) from the uterine wall Sweeping the membrane is another term for this.

Use a medication that can be placed directly in your vagina to soften and encourage your cervix to open. Because the cervical ripening process takes time, labor induction can take longer than spontaneous labor.

What are the various modes of delivery?

There are two types of deliveries: vaginal and cesarean (C-section). Your baby will pass naturally through the birth canal during vaginal birth. A C-section is a surgical procedure in which your provider makes an incision (cut) in your abdomen and the baby is delivered in an operating room. The most common type of birth is vaginal delivery. However, you may require a C-section for a variety of reasons, including:

- If your baby is not lying down with his or her head down,
- If your baby is too big to pass naturally through your pelvis,

- If your baby is in pain,

- If your cervix is blocked by the placenta (a condition called placenta previa),

- If you have health issues or complications that necessitate a C-section,

- If there is an emergency that necessitates the immediate delivery of your baby,

In many cases, a cesarean section is not decided until labor begins.

How long will I be hospitalized?

The length of your hospital stay will be determined by the hospital where you give birth and the type of delivery you have. Because a C-section is a surgical procedure, you will usually be in the hospital for a longer period. If you have any complications or health issues during your delivery, you may need to stay in the hospital for an extended period.

Conclusion

In this guide to what to expect during pregnancy, we have viewed and understand the trimesters and the changes you can expect as your pregnancy progresses.

Early warning signs Recognizing Early Warning Signs A missed menstrual cycle is one of the most common early signs of pregnancy.

Other than a missed period, signs of pregnancy may appear as early as the first few weeks of conception. Wearing a support bra and going up a bra size can make you feel more comfortable. Constipation is a result of the hormone progesterone slowing down the muscle contractions that move food through your system. Food cravings affect more than 60% of pregnant women. Your body is putting in a lot of effort to support a growing baby. Nausea is one of the most common complaints among expectant mothers.

For some pregnant women, the nausea is mild. Although your baby is still small, your uterus is expanding and putting pressure on your bladder. Respond as soon as possible when nature calls.

If you experience severe bleeding, cramping, or sharp pain in your abdomen, contact a doctor. Keep a healthy weight: "Eating for two" does not imply that a pregnant woman should eat twice as much.

Eat a healthy and balanced diet, which includes plenty of fruits, vegetables, and whole grains in reasonable portions.

Take vitamins and supplements exactly as directed by your doctor.

Drink plenty of fluids.

When you reach the second stage of labor, this is the stage of labor in which you will give birth to your baby.